The Cervical Solution

The Cervical Solution

Unspoken Fertility Info, Tips, & How-tos Every Woman Should Know

Ash Hernandez

I dedicate this book to the memory of my daughter Gwyneth, who passed away right before her life began in 2015. While I didn't get the opportunity to raise her or teach her about her female body like I had dreamed, her existence put me on a path of research and questioning. Gwyneth gave me the strength and courage I never imagined I could possess. Without her, this book would not have been possible.

Also, a big thank you to The Beautiful Cervix Project for the permission to use its real, raw, and extremely valuable cervix gallery images. Please visit https://www.beautifulcervix.com for more information and images of real-life cervixes!

Contents

Introduction

I'm so honored that you're here and about to embark on your natural fertility journey with *The Cervical Solution*!

Being a wife, mother of six, and a fertility coach has given me a deep appreciation for the cervix and its incredible yet rarely spoken about role in female fertility. I have avoided using hormonal birth control, IUDs, or any chemical contraception my entire life. My personal fertility journey, marked by years of observation, pregnancies, loss, and dedicated learning, has built an unshakeable confidence in my understanding and reverence for the reproductive cycle. I hold a handful of professional certifications, including Human Reproduction from the University of Adelaide, Advanced Training in Restorative Reproductive Medicine with NeoFertility, and am currently working towards a Fertility Education and Medical Management (FEMM) instructor certification at the end of 2025.

My goal for this book is to provide simple, succinct instructions for using your body, most specifically your cervix, to determine your fertile days. And, to provide these details to women of all ages so that over time, we will ALL be educated on how our bodies work. Being aware of our bodies' signs can allow us to achieve pregnancy faster, prevent pregnancy successfully, and determine if our hormones/menstrual cycle are working properly. Being familiar with our cervixes may also allow us to schedule medical consultations if unusual changes are noticed, complementing standard cervical cancer screenings like Pap smears and HPV tests.

The Cervical Solution, *TCS*, is NOT a guideline for sexual practices for the religious. ANY female, religious or not, can use this cervix-focused fertility awareness method. I can't stress that point enough. Oftentimes in society, churches, or on social media, Natural Family Planning (NFP)/ Fertility Awareness Methods (FAMS) are marketed to Christian and specifically Catholic audiences only, neglecting women of other religions who also deserve to understand and embrace their bodies. This book DOES NOT delve into artificial birth control, how it works, or arguments to convince you not to use it.

What this book WILL DO is give you a step-by-step breakdown on how to use your cervix and cervical mucus to track your fertile signs throughout your menstrual cycle. It is for ANY female who wants to understand her body, feel empowered by her discoveries, and enjoy either achieving or preventing pregnancy without side effects from birth control or the stress of full-time charting and temp-taking of other mainstream fertility awareness methods (FAM) or Natural Family Planning (NFP) methods.

The information in this book should be taught to ALL young women who are coming of age. In addition to learning how to put a condom on a banana in health class at school (something I'll always remember doing), girls should be learning the vital skill of tracking their fertility with the signs from their bodies.

It is outrageous to think that we walk around for most of our lives with such immense power within us, doing everything we can to push it down, turn it off, stop it! Then - when we're ready to finally use our fertility, it's malfunctioning, or we don't know how it works! As a mother, it is my job to ensure that my daughters confidently understand their reproductive systems so that they feel in control of the great power they hold within. I will also see to it that my sons are equipped with knowledge and respect for a woman's body as it transitions through the menstrual cycle.

Less of this! 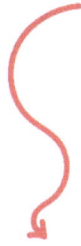 More of this!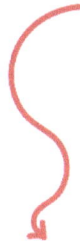

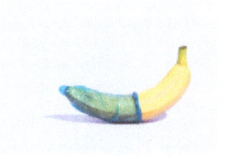 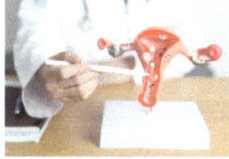

When I first told my two daughters, ages 7 and 9 that I was writing a book about *vaginas* they said, "Mommy, every girl who has a vagina knows how they work!" Cue the giggling and eye rolls.

But is that true? Do you know everything you should know about how your reproductive system works? Do you know how to find your cervix and what it feels like when fertile versus not fertile? If your answers are no, that's OK. You're here now and will soon have all the knowledge you need to successfully understand and optimize your fertility health.

I reached a point in my life when I realized that I didn't know much about my female body at all. It was in 2015, after I gave birth to my second daughter, Gwyneth, who tragically died shortly before she was born. I was completely overcome with grief for her lost life and grief for my fertility that I thought I had lost along with her. I desperately wanted to become pregnant again but realized I didn't know how to achieve that.

For my first 2 pregnancies, I had simply planned intercourse around day 14 (which we "hear" is the day of ovulation) and was fortunate enough to get pregnant right away. Since I had just given birth, I had no idea when my fertility would return or if this stillbirth would cause me to never have another child.

I decided it was time to start taking charge of my body, to understand why this stillbirth had occurred and how my menstrual cycle worked. I would later discover that Gwyneth had died from Prenatal Onset Group B Strep Disease. I'm forever grateful for the life lessons she taught me and how her death brought forth positivity in the form of my natural fertility journey, among other awakenings.

It's been 10 years since I began learning about how my body works and I am excited to share with you the knowledge I have acquired.

If you have been wanting to stop using hormonal birth control or chemical contraceptives but are too nervous to give it a try, this book is for YOU!

If you are trying to boost your chances of conceiving, this book is for YOU! If you are trying to prevent pregnancy right now, this book is also for YOU!

This method is SUPER straightforward but, I'm not going to lie and tell you that zero work is involved. I will be honest - a woman's fertility, our ability to bring life into this world is an AMAZING gift. Society doesn't teach us to appreciate that from a young age. We are taught that it's a burden and given ways to immediately halt our fertility during our most fertile years! The ability to achieve pregnancy is a power that we have no choice but to embrace and learn to tame.

As the Spider-Man saying goes, "With great power comes great responsibility." And *that* is the truth about a woman's fertility.

There have been many times when I sat crying, overwhelmed by the heavy weight of being the carrier and birther of life for my growing family. But as I learned how to interpret my cervix to decipher my fertility, and as my childbearing years are quickly flying by, I've realized how precious and fleeting our fertile time is. I hope after reading this book, you will feel the same!

The two key resources that helped me tremendously to understand my own body during the last 10 years were the book *Taking Charge of Your Fertility* by Toni Weschler and the website *The Beautiful Cervix Project,* www.beautifulcervix.com. Both provided me with a great starting point for understanding what should happen to my body and cervix and when it should happen during my cycle.

Please note that I am not a medical professional. If you have medical issues or questions, please seek a physician for all medical advice. My knowledge derives from my multiple certifications, my own research, and experiences practicing fertility awareness myself for over a decade. Since I have never altered my cycle with anything other than pregnancy and breastfeeding, I have been able to experience my reproductive signs as straightforward. Every woman has a different health and medical history that could lead to varying or unusual signs and symptoms during the menstrual cycle.

What is the Fertility Awareness Method (FAM)?

TCS is a type of fertility awareness. To begin, let's first break down what FAM is and what it can help you do.

Fertility Awareness Method (FAM) encompasses natural family planning approaches that involve tracking various fertility signs. This information is used to determine a woman's fertile and infertile phases within her menstrual cycle. It empowers women to understand how their reproductive system works and make informed decisions about contraception, achieving pregnancy, or managing reproductive health.

Key components often included in Fertility Awareness Methods include:

- **Basal Body Temperature (BBT):** This method involves taking daily measurements of basal body temperature upon waking up in the morning before engaging in any activity. A sustained rise in basal body temperature typically indicates that ovulation has already occurred, primarily due to increased progesterone levels (Mayo Clinic, 2023; StatPearls, n.d.-a).

- **Cervical Position & Mucus Observation:** Changes in cervical position and mucus consistency and appearance can help identify the fertile window (Leão & Esteves, 2024; Medical News Today, 2024; myFertileDays, n.d.; Taunton et al., 2014). As estrogen rises during the follicular phase, it has a profound impact on the cervix. It causes it to soften, rise high, and open the cervical os. After ovulation has occurred, estrogen decreases, causing the cervix to become dry, lower its position, and close the os. Fertile cervical mucus, which becomes clear, stretchy, and slippery around ovulation due to rising estrogen, also indicates the fertile period is approaching or present.

- **Calendar Tracking:** Tracking menstrual cycles on a calendar provides a general overview of cycle length and predicts the timing of ovulation based on past patterns. However, this method alone is less reliable than methods tracking physiological signs like mucus or temperature, especially for women with irregular cycles (Cleveland Clinic, n.d.-b; NHS, 2024).

FAM can be used for:

- **Contraception:** By avoiding unprotected intercourse during fertile days, couples can use FAMs as a natural method of contraception. Effectiveness varies depending on the method used and how well it is adhered to. Perfect use effectiveness for some methods can be up to 99%, but typical use effectiveness, reflecting real-world use, is lower, ranging roughly from 76-88% (Medical News Today, 2024; NHS, 2024). Diligent tracking and adherence are crucial if you want to trust and rely on FAM for contraception (Medical News Today, 2024; NHS, 2024).

- **Achieving Pregnancy:** For couples trying to conceive, FAM helps identify the most fertile days within the menstrual cycle, increasing the chances of successful conception (Medical News Today, 2024; myFertileDays, n.d.). We no longer have to time intercourse around Day 14 of the cycle. We know that women can ovulate early or later in the cycle, so simply aiming for Day 14th may not always lead to conception for every woman.

- **Reproductive Health Monitoring:** FAM encourages awareness of menstrual cycle regularity and provides insights into reproductive health. Changes in fertility signs may indicate hormonal imbalances, ovulatory disorders, or other underlying health conditions requiring medical evaluation (Cleveland Clinic, 2022; myFertileDays, n.d.). Checking your cervical position allows you to feel the cervical os and note if the tissue feels painful, unhealthy, etc. and get to a medical professional for further examinations.

What's Different about *TCS* vs. other FAMs?

TCS utilizes the cervix - its positioning within the body and the state of the cervical os, along with its mucus - as a primary focus for determining fertile vs. infertile phases. In other FAMs, cervical position is often presented as an optional or secondary sign, whereas TCS emphasizes its importance.

Another significant difference is that this method is symptom-hormonal and doesn't rely on Basal Body Temperature (BBT.) This is because I personally found BBT challenging to measure consistently and interpret accurately amidst the demands of daily life. To track BBT effectively, one needs to take her temperature at the exact same time every morning before any activity, using a sensitive and appropriate thermometer, and chart the readings daily over months to establish a pattern (Cleveland Clinic, n.d.-b; Mayo Clinic, 2023; StatPearls, n.d.-a).

Normally, a woman's BBT is slightly lower in the first half of the cycle -follicular phase and rises after ovulation due to increased progesterone - luteal phase (Mayo Clinic, 2023; StatPearls, n.d.-a). A sustained rise in BBT (typically 0.5 to 1.0°F or 0.3 to 0.6°C) indicates ovulation has likely taken place (Mayo Clinic, 2023; StatPearls, n.d.-a). However, accurate BBT tracking requires consistent, precise measurements immediately upon waking, and readings can be affected by factors like illness, stress, sleep disturbances, or alcohol (Cleveland Clinic, n.d.-b; Mayo Clinic, 2023; StatPearls, n.d.-a). If I ran off to attend to a crying child first thing upon waking (which I'm sure you know is common!) and missed taking my temperature, the data for that day would be unreliable. Furthermore, BBT confirms ovulation retrospectively; it shows when ovulation has *already* occurred, it does not predict it prospectively (Cleveland Clinic, n.d.-b; Mayo Clinic, 2023).

While BBT can be a useful indicator when used correctly, particularly in combination with other signs (like in the sympto-thermal method,) its perceived difficulty and retrospective nature led to its exclusion from the core *TCS* method described here. It felt much easier for me to assess my cervix's position and openness, which can be done any time of day, not only upon waking. Therefore, I eventually focused solely on the cervix and its mucus.

Another difference is that many FAMs incorporate algorithms or calculations based on past cycle data to predict the fertile window (Cleveland Clinic, n.d.-b). *TCS* emphasizes observing your *own* body's signs in the *present* moment to determine your current fertility status. There is minimal guessing or predicting involved based on averages. While looking back at previous cycles helps confirm patterns, the primary focus is on interpreting the signs your body is showing *now*. This is important because factors such as stress, illness, and travel can affect cycle length and ovulation timing, causing variations from month to month (Cleveland Clinic, n.d.-b; Medical News Today, 2024). Every cycle can be slightly different, and observing present signs provides the most immediate insight.

Lastly - the cost of this method is extremely low compared to other approaches. Some FAM programs involve fees for long term instructors or require specific Clear Blue monitoring devices and coordinating test strips, potentially costing hundreds of dollars initially or ongoing (Simcha, Fischer, 2020). I feel strongly that such vital information about female body's should be accessible to all women, regardless of financial status. That's why this book is priced affordably, and the necessary supplies are nominal.

I don't support gatekeeping of information that makes such a huge impact on a woman's life and wellbeing. I'm here to educate you and provide guidance as needed for minimal costs. Once you understand how your unique body changes during your cycle, you **really can** track your fertility naturally and you won't need me! My goal is to teach you what to look for in your own body so that you rely on and trust **yourself**, not **me**, to monitor your fertility. Being a fertility coach allows me to support women in whatever way they need it on their journeys. However, the best thing you can do is take this knowledge, apply it to your body / relationship, and go on to live a stress-free, empowered, and independent life. The ultimate goal is for women to no longer fear their fertility or view it as a heavy burden, but to embrace the amazing gift that it is, once they are educated on how it functions.

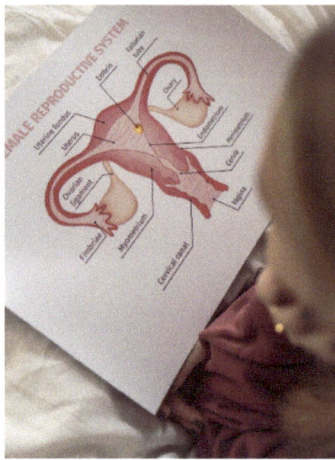

Why does *TCS* focus on the Cervix?

TCS is a sympto-hormonal form of FAM. That means the method focuses on monitoring cervical mucus and urine metabolites. Sympto-thermal methods look at many different fertility signs, which gives us the most extensive view of our fertility. I don't know about you, but I'm the type of person who wants to have **ALL** the details and gather **ALL** the knowledge before making my decisions.

That's why I love sympto-thermal and sympto-hormonal FAM and why I created *TCS*! *TCS* makes the cervix the focus of the plan because of how dramatic the changes to it are, and how reliable it is once you know what you're feeling. The cervix is essentially the door to the female reproductive system.

The cervix is the lower, narrow part of the uterus that opens into the vagina (Cleveland Clinic, 2022). It has a generally cylindrical shape and is composed of various tissues, including:

- **External Os:** This is the opening of the cervix into the vagina (Cleveland Clinic, 2022). It can dilate significantly during childbirth, and dilates slightly throughout your cycle to allow for sperm entry and blood to exit.

- **Cervical Canal:** This passageway connects the internal os (opening into the uterus) to the external os (Cleveland Clinic, 2022).

- **Cervical Glands:** These glands secrete mucus, which plays a vital role in protecting the uterus and influencing sperm transport (myFertileDays, n.d.; Taunton et al., 2014).

The structure and position of the cervix are dynamic, undergoing changes throughout the menstrual cycle in response to hormonal fluctuations (myFertileDays, n.d.; Reed & Carr, 2024). The cervical os changes in openness around ovulation, as it opens for sperm to move through, then closes slowly after ovulation has occurred. (myFertileDays, n.d.; Reed & Carr, 2024). It is also responsible for dilating dramatically to the infamous "10 centimeters" during vaginal childbirth and then returning to its non-pregnant state. It is quite an astonishing organ!

Since the release of this book in 2024, I have spoken to many women to personally get their reviews and reactions to the concept of "finding" their cervix. I'm a girl who's "not afraid to get her hands dirty," as they say. However, some women are….and here's the thing….this method pushes you to get over the reluctance of exploring your own body. We owe it to ourselves and to our families now and in the future, to be educated. Knowledge can change the future for women in so many positive ways. Especially living in modern times, during times of political unrest and evolving laws and rights, we must always remember **this** – no one can take away our fertility knowledge; our body literacy. And it's something that can be passed on for generations to come. We may have to do some meticulous research and tracking, but the reward will be worth all the hard work. I have experienced it firsthand and am doing my part to spread the word.

Various Cervical Positions You Feel & When

The position of the cervix changes throughout the menstrual cycle due to hormonal (estrogen) fluctuations (myFertileDays, n.d.; Reed & Carr, 2024). Here's an overview of the typical changes in cervical position:

- **Low Cervix:** During menstruation and the early follicular phase, when estrogen levels are low, the cervix tends to be positioned lower in the vaginal canal. It may feel firm and relatively closed, with the cervical os only slightly open to allow menstrual blood to flow. In my experience, the cervical os is open so slightly that you may not even believe that blood could flow out of it, but just that little slit of an opening is enough for menstruation. If you've ever had intercourse during this phase of your cycle, you may find it a bit uncomfortable, even painful, as if a wall is preventing full penetration. Well, that "wall" is the cervix in a lower position in your body.

- **Medium Cervix:** Between the low and high positions, the cervix may be in a medium position during the mid-follicular and mid-luteal phases of the menstrual cycle. It is not as low as during menstruation nor as high as during ovulation.

- **High Cervix:** As ovulation approaches (late follicular phase), rising estrogen levels cause the cervix to rise higher in the vaginal canal. Around ovulation, the cervix is typically at its highest position. The days leading up to ovulation will have the cervix climbing higher and higher. It will be more difficult to reach, and you will notice you'll need to insert your finger further up into your vaginal canal, perhaps to your second knuckle. It will feel softer and more open, with the cervical os dilated to facilitate sperm entry into the uterus. If you've ever had intercourse during your fertile days, you may have noticed that there is no "wall" and that full penetration is possible due to the high cervix, allowing the sperm to get as close to the cervical os as possible.

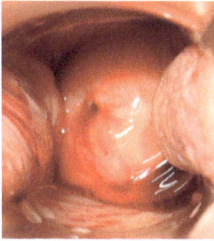

Low Cervix

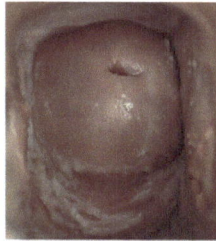

Medium Cervix

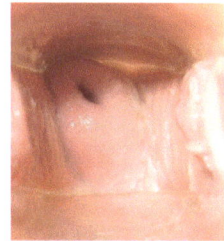

High Cervix

The goal of monitoring your cervix with *TCS* is to follow the changes in the cervix. Finding it:

- initially slightly open after your period ends,

- proceeding to wide open leading up to and at ovulation,

- and then proceeding to closed once again near the end of your cycle.

Cervical Mucus & its Role in Fertility

Cervical mucus plays an important role in fertility and reproductive health (Leão & Esteves, 2024; myFertileDays, n.d.; Taunton et al., 2014). Its composition and consistency change significantly throughout the menstrual cycle under hormonal influence (primarily estrogen and progesterone), facilitating or inhibiting sperm transport based on its consistency (Leão & Esteves, 2024; myFertileDays, n.d.; Taunton et al., 2014).

Cervical mucus is primarily composed of water, electrolytes, proteins (mucins), carbohydrates, and various enzymes. Under the influence of rising estrogen before ovulation, cervical mucus becomes abundant, thin, clear, and stretchy (often compared to raw egg whites) – this is considered fertile mucus (Leão & Esteves, 2024; myFertileDays, n.d.; Taunton et al., 2014). After ovulation, rising progesterone causes mucus to become thicker, tackier, and less permeable to sperm (myFertileDays, n.d.; Taunton et al., 2014).

The thin, watery, stretchy consistency of fertile mucus provides an optimal alkaline environment (pH ~7.0-8.5) that protects sperm from the acidic vagina (pH ~3.8-4.5) and aids sperm motility and transport through the cervix towards the uterus and fallopian tubes (Leão & Esteves, 2024; myFertileDays, n.d.; Taunton et al., 2014).

Mucus for Trying to Avoid (TTA) or NOT Achieve pregnancy. Usually seen after ovulation occurs and up until period begins.

Infertile quality (thick, tacky) cervical mucus

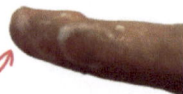

Fertile quality (clear, stretchy) cervical mucus

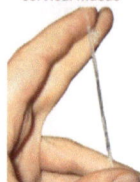

Ideal mucus for Trying to Conceive (TTC) but NOT "go time" if you are Trying to Avoid (TTA).

Understanding Your Menstrual Cycle

Menstruation: The cycle begins on Day 1, the first day of true menstrual bleeding. At the beginning of the menstrual cycle, several ovarian follicles start to develop under the influence of Follicle-Stimulating Hormone (FSH) produced by the pituitary gland (Reed & Carr, 2024). Each follicle contains an immature egg. During menstruation, the uterine lining (endometrium) is shed. The cervix is typically low and firm, with the os slightly open to allow blood to flow out (myFertileDays, n.d.; Reed & Carr, 2024).

Follicular Phase: Following menstruation, estrogen levels begin to rise as follicles develop. One follicle typically becomes dominant and continues to grow while the others regress (Reed & Carr, 2024). Rising estrogen stimulates the rebuilding of the endometrium (Reed & Carr, 2024). As estrogen levels rise leading up to ovulation, the cervix begins to soften, rise, and open slightly (myFertileDays, n.d.; Reed & Carr, 2024). Cervical mucus increases in quantity and becomes clearer and more elastic, resembling raw egg whites (Leão & Esteves, 2024; myFertileDays, n.d.; Reed & Carr, 2024; Taunton et al., 2014). Around the middle of the cycle, a surge in luteinizing hormone (LH) triggers the final maturation and release of the egg from the dominant follicle (ovulation), typically 24-36 hours after the surge begins (Reed & Carr, 2024).

Ovulation: This is the event where the mature egg is released from the dominant follicle (Reed & Carr, 2024). At peak fertility around ovulation, the cervix is typically high, soft, and open (myFertileDays, n.d.; Reed & Carr, 2024). Cervical mucus is abundant, slippery, and transparent ('egg white' quality), facilitating sperm transport (Leão & Esteves, 2024; myFertileDays, n.d.; Reed & Carr, 2024; Taunton et al., 2014). The released egg is viable for fertilization for about 12-24 hours (Cleveland Clinic, n.d.-b).

Luteal Phase: After ovulation, the ruptured follicle transforms into the corpus luteum, which produces progesterone (Reed & Carr, 2024). Progesterone prepares the uterine lining for potential implantation of a fertilized egg and causes characteristic changes in fertility signs. The cervix begins to lower, firm up, and close (myFertileDays, n.d.; Reed & Carr, 2024). Cervical mucus decreases in quantity and becomes stickier, thicker, and cloudier as progesterone levels rise (Leão & Esteves, 2024; myFertileDays, n.d.; Reed & Carr, 2024; Taunton et al., 2014). Basal body temperature also rises slightly due to progesterone (Mayo Clinic, 2023; StatPearls, n.d.-a). If pregnancy does not occur, the corpus luteum degrades, progesterone and estrogen levels fall, triggering the shedding of the uterine lining (menstruation), and the cycle begins again with a period (Reed & Carr, 2024).

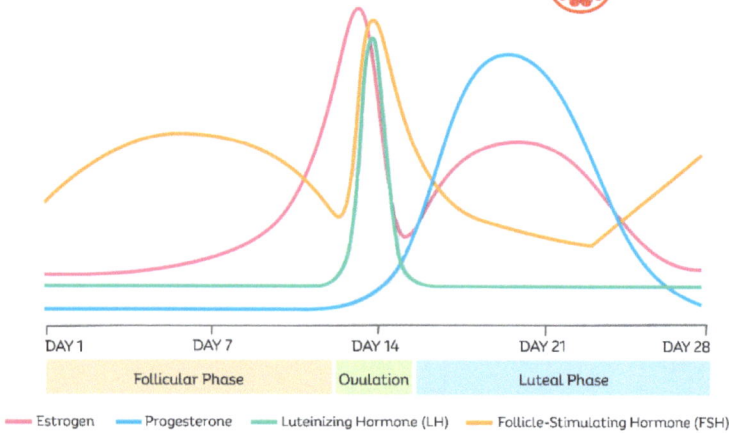

HORMONE FLUCTUATIONS OF THE MENSTRUAL CYCLE

DAY 1 — DAY 7 — DAY 14 — DAY 21 — DAY 28

Follicular Phase | Ovulation | Luteal Phase

Estrogen | Progesterone | Luteinizing Hormone (LH) | Follicle-Stimulating Hormone (FSH)

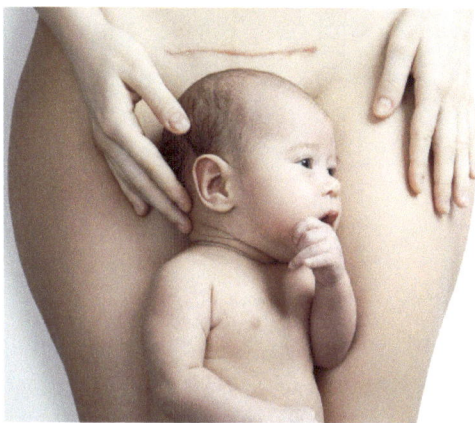

The Ever Elusive…Postpartum

If you've delivered a baby, then you're familiar with the confusing and often erratic postpartum months following your vaginal delivery or c-section. Hormonal shifts can cause a rollercoaster of physical and emotional changes. Exhaustion and initially low libido are normal and common. You might observe fertile-looking cervical mucus, then dryness, then fertile mucus again – what is going on?! As libido potentially returns, questions arise: Where am I, fertility-wise? Is it true that breastfeeding is natural birth control? Am I ready to conceive again? Or do I want to avoid another pregnancy soon after birth?

So how do you determine your fertility status during that tricky postpartum period? The answer involves careful observation, again, with a focus on your cervix! Continue monitoring your cervix and mucus using *TCS* method instructions, understanding that patterns will likely be irregular initially.

Immediately after birth, you will experience lochia – the postpartum discharge of blood, mucus, and uterine tissue, typically lasting 4-8 weeks. Following this, if you are breastfeeding, you may experience a period of amenorrhea (no periods) and potentially less cervical mucus.

Eventually, you will notice patches of fertile-quality mucus appearing and disappearing as your body attempts to resume ovulation. Predicting the *first* postpartum ovulation with certainty is difficult, but observing your signs provides clues.

- **No fertile mucus, closed cervix:** Likely indicates lower fertility.

- **Increasing fertile mucus, closed cervix:** Indicates potential fertility. Your body is showing signs of estrogen activity, but ovulation might still be weeks or months away. However, the presence of fertile mucus means conception is possible if ovulation occurs unexpectedly.

- **Increasing fertile mucus, opening/open cervix:** Strongly suggests fertility has returned and ovulation is near or occurring.

Remember: Using progesterone test strips (like Proov) or a Mira Hormone monitor, after a suspected ovulation can help confirm if ovulation occurred by detecting the post-ovulatory rise in progesterone. If no rise is detected despite fertile signs, ovulation likely **did not** happen, and you remain potentially fertile.

Your first few cycles after giving birth can be irregular – shorter, longer, heavier, lighter than your pre-pregnancy norm. This is why observing your *current* signs with *TCS* is so valuable.

To address the breastfeeding birth control question: Yes, full time breastfeeding can prevent fertility from returning under specific conditions known as the **Lactational Amenorrhea Method (LAM)** (Singh et al., 2018; UNC School of Medicine, n.d.; Van der Wijden & Manheimer, 1998; UC Davis Health, 2023). If you are breastfeeding exclusively or almost exclusively (meaning the baby receives little to no other food or liquids, nursing frequently day and night with no long intervals, often without pacifiers), AND your menstrual periods have *not* returned, AND your baby is less than six months old, LAM can be highly effective (over 98% effective against pregnancy) (NHS, 2024; Singh et al., 2018; Van der Wijden & Manheimer, 1998; UC Davis Health, 2023). If *any* of these three conditions are not met (e.g., periods return, you supplement feedings regularly, baby starts solids, baby sleeps through the night consistently, baby is older than 6 months), LAM is no longer considered reliable, and another contraceptive method or abstaining should be used if pregnancy is not desired (NHS, 2024; Van der Wijden & Manheimer, 1998). I have found this aligns with my personal experience; my cycle typically returned around 12 months postpartum. I have breastfed all my babies on demand and co-sleep until about 12 months. Around this time is when babies become more interested in solid foods and sleeping, that's when I see my menstrual cycle return.

The postpartum months before your period returns can be challenging. You may feel overwhelmed by mothering a newborn, dealing with sleep deprivation, and feeling pressure to resume intercourse. You might feel unprepared or anxious about conceiving again soon. Irish twins do happen! Always listen to your body and your feelings; never feel guilty about waiting to resume intimacy until you feel physically and emotionally ready. The common "6-week checkup" clearance is a guideline, not a mandate for resuming intercourse. Communicate with your partner about your needs and timeline. For me, pausing sexual activity for a period after birth helped reduce stress and allowed for healing. That is perfectly okay. Partners may need you to communicate this to them. Don't hesitate to let your partner know how you are feeling and work on trying to strengthen your relationship in other ways beyond intercourse. I know…easier said than done, but in the end, it's worth it - for your body and your relationship.

In my experience, when I was ready to resume and meticulously followed *TCS* plan – monitoring the cervix and avoiding intercourse when the cervix showed any signs of opening or fertile mucus was present – this helped me prevent pregnancy. Conversely, if I engaged in intercourse when potentially fertile signs were present or I hadn't confirmed ovulation had occurred and passed, I successfully conceived.

As an active FAM/NFP user and advocate, I am a part of many social media groups and accounts pertaining to the methods. I have witnessed a multitude of women really struggling during the postpartum period. Many women become overwhelmed and confused by their fertility and find themselves unintentionally pregnant again, soon after a recent pregnancy. This is a time when we need to be as diligent as possible in monitoring the cervix. If you are seriously TTA, I recommend always doing a cervical check prior to engaging in intercourse. If you feel the os softening, raising, and opening, you can confirm that you **must** refrain at this time. So many difficult and stressful method failure pregnancies could be spaced more appropriately if women understood the importance of a quick cervical check. I don't know of any other FAMs that encourage you to do this "safety" check. In my opinion, with my knowledge of the cervix, this is a no-brainer. There is no reason to be "in the dark" regarding your fertility status; especially when we have the cervix!

With *TCS* as your guide, you can better navigate postpartum fertility based on your goals, using your cervix and cervical mucus observations. Avoid guessing and taking "heat of the moment" risks, as that increases the risk of an unintended outcome.

Movement for Fertility

Alongside diet, your physical activity habits play a significant role in shaping your menstrual cycle, fertility signs, and overall reproductive health. How you move your body can influence hormonal balance, ovulation regularity, stress levels. Here I am highlighting the benefits of balanced physical activity and the potential pitfalls of too much or too little, so that you have an optimal approach for supporting a healthy menstrual cycle. Whether you are Trying to Conceive (TTC) or Trying to Avoid (TTA) you want your fertility to be functioning properly.

Exercise can help regulate hormones, including insulin, which is crucial for ovulation (Reproductive Science Center of New Jersey, n.d.). Exercise increases the body's sensitivity to insulin making it available to use for energy, faster. Too much insulin in the bloodstream can cause eggs to stop maturing and therefore interfere with successful ovulation. This is particularly beneficial for women with conditions like Polycystic Ovary Syndrome (PCOS), where insulin resistance is common and can cause anovulation. Physical activity is also a great stress reliever, and chronic stress can negatively impact reproductive hormones.

While moderate exercise is beneficial for the body and specifically the reproductive system, too much intense exercise can have the opposite effect. Overtraining or engaging in very strenuous workouts, particularly without adequate calories to match the energy expenditure, can place significant stress on the body. If you're consistently burning significantly more calories than you're consuming, this tells the body you're in a time of famine. In such situations, to conserve energy for essential survival functions, it may shut down non-essential processes like your menstrual cycle.

Too much exercise can also lead to a disruption of the Hypothalamic-Pituitary-Ovarian (HPO) Axis. This is the delicate hormonal communication pathway between your brain (hypothalamus and pituitary gland) and your ovaries that controls your menstrual cycle. Excessive physical stress can suppress the signals from the hypothalamus, leading to irregular periods, anovulation (lack of ovulation), or functional hypothalamic amenorrhea (the absence of menstruation due to non-organic causes) (Reproductive Science Center of New Jersey, n.d.; Uni ScholarWorks, n.d.).This is often seen in female athletes and causes them low energy and low bone density, and low levels of body fat, often a result of intense training and restrictive dieting. This can impair estrogen production, as fat tissue contributes to estrogen synthesis. Insufficient estrogen can further contribute to menstrual irregularities and anovulation.

However, a complete lack of physical activity can also negatively impact fertility. A life of no exercise can contribute to weight gain, potential obesity, and insulin resistance. So, what's the perfect amount of exercise? The general recommendation for adults, including those trying to conceive, is at least 150 minutes of moderate-intensity aerobic exercise per week. Examples include brisk walking, cycling at a moderate pace, swimming, or dancing. Alternatively, 75 minutes of vigorous-intensity aerobic exercise per week, or an equivalent combination of moderate and vigorous activity, is also recommended (Reproductive Science Center of New Jersey, n.d.).

Be sure to include muscle-strengthening activities that work all major muscle groups (legs, hips, back, abdomen, chest, shoulders, and arms) on 2 or more days a week. This helps build lean muscle mass, which can improve metabolism and insulin sensitivity (Genesis OBGYN, n.d.). Even 15 minutes of lifting light dumbbells will improve your cycle.

- **Listen to Your Body:** This is the most crucial advice. Pay attention to signs of overtraining, such as persistent fatigue that isn't relieved by rest, changes in your menstrual cycle (e.g., periods becoming irregular or stopping), recurrent injuries, mood disturbances, or a decline in exercise performance. If you're new to exercise, start slowly and gradually increase intensity and duration. Yoga and Pilates are excellent choices as they not only improve flexibility, core strength, and balance but are also renowned for their stress-reducing benefits.

If you have any underlying health conditions, a history of eating disorders, or are unsure about what type or amount of exercise is appropriate for you while trying to conceive, it is always best to consult with your healthcare provider or a qualified exercise physiologist.

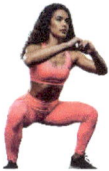

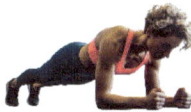

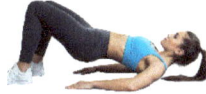

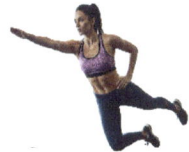

Exercise	Type	Focus Area	Notes & Tips
Squats	Strength Training	Glutes, Hamstrings, Quadriceps, Core	Keep your chest up, back straight, and push through your heels. Imagine sitting back into a chair.
Plank	Pilates/Strength	Core (Abs, Obliques, Lower Back), Shoulders	Maintain a straight line from head to heels. Engage your core and avoid sagging your hips.
Glute Bridge	Pilates/Strength	Glutes, Hamstrings, Core	Squeeze your glutes at the top of the movement. Keep your neck relaxed and lift through your hips.
Bird-Dog	Pilates/Strength	Core Stability, Balance, Back	Move slowly and with control. Keep your core engaged to prevent rocking your torso. Extend opposite arm and leg.

Nourishment for Fertility

Beyond understanding the direct signals your cervix and cervical mucus provide, it's empowering to recognize how your dietary choices can profoundly influence your menstrual cycle, fertility signs, and overall reproductive health. What you eat impacts hormonal balance, ovulation regularity, the quality of your cervical mucus, and even your ability to conceive and maintain a healthy pregnancy.

Your body requires a steady supply of nutrients to perform all its complex functions, including those essential for reproduction. A well-balanced diet provides everything you need for hormone production, healthy egg development, and a uterus ready for implantation.

When we're young we can afford to eat some junk food here and there, drink alcohol at a party, and not exercise the next day. But as we age and especially if we're in a period where we're trying to conceive a healthy baby, women need to be mindful of the correlation between our lifestyles and our menstrual cycles.

One of the simplest yet most crucial aspects of a fertility-friendly diet is adequate hydration. Water is fundamental to nearly every bodily process, and its role in reproductive health is no exception. In regards to your fertility signs, hydration directly impacts the quality and quantity of your cervical mucus. Being dehydrated affects all of your mucus membranes. If you are not drinking enough water, your cervical mucus can become thicker, stickier, and less abundant (Cleveland Clinic, n.d.-c). Fertile-quality cervical mucus, which is typically thin, watery, and stretchy like egg whites, creates an ideal environment for sperm to survive and travel towards the egg. Dehydration can hinder sperm motility and survival (Stony Brook Medicine, n.d.). Your goal is to drink plenty of water throughout the day – aiming for around 8-10 glasses (or 2-2.75 liters) depending on your activity level and climate.

In addition to getting enough water, a diet rich in whole, unprocessed food provides all the nutrients your reproductive system needs. Choose whole grains like oats, quinoa, brown rice, and whole-wheat bread over refined carbohydrates (white bread, pastries, sugary cereals). Complex carbohydrates are digested more slowly, helping to maintain stable blood sugar and insulin levels. Like much of the advice in this book, these changes in diet and habits may not be easy right away. I've been right where you may be, looking at my diet, thinking, "I don't eat *that* bad…" But once I looked in depth at my diet, there was lots of room for improvement. And that's what you must do to begin. Start with small areas of improvement and make changes slowly.

Adequate protein is essential for egg and sperm development. While animal protein is a source, studies suggest that replacing some animal proteins (especially red and processed meats) with plant-based proteins like beans, lentils, nuts, seeds, and tofu may be beneficial for fertility (Gaskins & Chavarro, 2018; Panth et al., 2018). If you are able, purchase meat from local farms that feed grass-only and do not vaccinate animals with antibiotics that will then be passed on to the humans who eat them.

Monounsaturated fats (found in avocados, olive oil, nuts) and polyunsaturated fats, particularly omega-3 fatty acids (found in fatty fish like salmon, flaxseeds, chia seeds, and walnuts), are crucial for hormone production, reducing inflammation, and supporting overall reproductive health (Gaskins & Chavarro, 2018; Panth et al., 2018). Trans fats, "bad fats," often found in processed and fried foods, have been linked to an increased risk of ovulatory infertility and should be avoided (Gaskins & Chavarro, 2018).

There are a core group of vitamins that are important for successful ovulation and conception. First - Folic Acid (Folate): B-vitamin is critical for preventing neural tube defects in a developing baby. Beyond that, adequate folate intake has been associated with improved fertility because it lowers the risk of anovulation (Gaskins & Chavarro, 2018; Panth et al., 2018). Good sources include leafy green vegetables (spinach, kale), legumes, asparagus, and fortified grains.

Second is iron. Iron deficiency can potentially lead to anovulation. Eating iron-rich foods is important. You can get iron from plant-based sources - beans, lentils, spinach, and fortified cereals. Consuming with a source of Vitamin C (to aid absorption) may be particularly beneficial for fertility, in addition to iron from red meat.

Third is Vitamin D: Emerging research suggests Vitamin D plays a role in female reproduction, including ovarian function and implantation. Sunlight exposure and foods like fatty fish and fortified dairy or plant milks are sources.

Fourth is Antioxidants (Vitamins C & E, Selenium, Zinc): These compounds help protect your eggs (and sperm, for your partner) from damage caused by oxidative stress. Colorful fruits and vegetables (berries, citrus fruits, bell peppers), nuts, seeds, and whole grains are packed with antioxidants (Panth et al., 2018; Reproductive Science Center, n.d.-b).

We have all heard this time and time again, but it can never hurt to go through another reminder of what we should minimize and avoid in our diets! We should aim to avoid processed foods, added sugars, and trans fats. As mentioned, these can negatively impact insulin levels, promote inflammation, and contribute to weight gain, all of which can impair fertility.

If you're trying to conceive, now's a good time to look at your caffeine intake and reduce it if possible. The relationship between caffeine and fertility is complex, but high intake (generally over 200-300 milligrams per day, equivalent to about two to three 8-ounce cups of coffee) has been associated in some studies with a longer time to achieve pregnancy and an increased risk of miscarriage (Texas Fertility Center, n.d.; Your

Fertility, 2018).

We all know this - limit or remove alcohol from our diets to improve our fertility health. Alcohol consumption can negatively affect fertility in several ways: disrupting ovulation and hormonal balance and decreasing fecundability (the probability of conceiving in each menstrual cycle) according to some studies (Kesmodel et al., 2002). The American College of Obstetricians and Gynecologists (ACOG, 2021) advises that there is no known safe amount of alcohol use during pregnancy or while trying to get pregnant. It's generally recommended to limit or avoid alcohol when actively trying to conceive or if you're experiencing irregular cycles.

A personal experience recently proved to me that our dietary choices are powerful factors that can significantly influence our menstrual cycles and our overall reproductive well-being. I have always liked to be on the go, not a big watcher of TV, and *never* sat down on the couch ever during the busy days with my kids. However, up until this year, I never went to the gym, lifted weights, or even went on consistent walks. When I turned 38, I started to feel tired and lethargic upon waking in the morning. I noticed my period getting heavier and irregular - both shorter and longer. And - the worst was that my hair began to thin and fall out! I felt like I was 4 months postpartum with all my hair loss, yet I WASN'T! After a visit to the doctor, some research and pondering over my diet and lifestyle, I decided to begin regular exercise and strength training 7 days a week. I started light Pilates workouts with dumbbells. I removed all candy, alcohol, cereals, and desserts. I began eating protein rich eggs for breakfast daily. I was shocked at how drastically my symptoms improved! Every negative symptom was gone after about 3 weeks of consistent exercise and a diet focusing on hydration, limited sugar, and higher proteins. I kept telling my husband, "It's amazing how, if we put good things into our bodies, good things happen. Everything works properly and we feel good!" It's such a simple concept, but with the stress and chaos of life, we may not always be fueling our bodies with the best foods.

By focusing on a balanced, whole-foods diet rich in essential nutrients, staying well-hydrated, and making exercise a natural part of your daily routine, you can actively support your body's natural fertility.

Remember, every woman's body is unique and amazing. Our bodies CAN change and heal, if we make the corrections needed. While these general guidelines are based on scientific evidence, it's always best to listen to your own body's signals. If you have specific concerns about your diet or fertility, don't hesitate to consult with your healthcare provider or a registered dietitian specializing in fertility. Taking these proactive steps can empower you on your journey towards achieving your reproductive goals.

Leafy Greens	Spinach, kale	Rich in folate, crucial for egg health.
Fatty Fish	Salmon, sardines	Omega-3s may regulate hormones, improve blood flow.
Berries	Blueberries, raspberries	Antioxidants protect eggs, reduce inflammation.
Legumes	Lentils, beans	High in protein, fiber, folate; may improve ovulation.
Whole Grains	Oats, quinoa	Complex carbs, fiber aid blood sugar, hormone balance.
Nuts & Seeds	Walnuts, flaxseeds	Healthy fats, vitamin E, zinc support reproductive health.
Full-Fat Dairy	Whole milk, Greek yogurt	Calcium, vitamin D, fats may improve ovulatory function.
Lean Proteins	Poultry, fish, eggs	Important for hormone production, cell function. Eggs offer choline.
Colorful Produce	Bell peppers, sweet potatoes	Vitamins, minerals, antioxidants support overall reproductive function.
Avocados		Monounsaturated fats, folate support hormone regulation.

Hidden Influencers: Endocrine Disruptors

In our "artificial" world, whether we're aware of it or not, we're surrounded by a vast lineup of synthetic chemicals every single day. While these products serve various purposes, some contain substances known as endocrine disruptors (EDs). These compounds can interfere with our body's delicate hormonal balance, potentially impacting the menstrual cycle, fertility signs, and overall reproductive health. Understanding Eds, what they are, where they're commonly found, and how they can affect your hormonal system, is an important aspect of taking a comprehensive approach to your reproductive well-being. I'm including this chapter because this falls under the category of "UNSPOKEN - things no one tells us is affecting our fertility…"

The endocrine system is a complex network of glands (like the ovaries, thyroid, pituitary, and adrenal glands) that produce and release hormones. These hormones act as chemical messengers, traveling through the bloodstream to regulate a vast array of bodily functions, including growth and development, metabolism, mood, sleep, and, crucially, reproduction (Endocrine Society, n.d.; National Institute of Environmental Health Sciences [NIEHS], n.d.-a). EDs are exogenous substances. This means they originate outside the body and can interfere with any aspect of hormone function. They can:

- Mimic natural hormones: Some EDs have structures like natural hormones (estrogen or testosterone) and can bind to hormone receptors in cells, tricking the body into responding as if a natural hormone were present, often at inappropriate times or in excessive amounts (Endocrine Society, n.d.; Diamanti-Kandarakis et al., 2009).

- Block natural hormones: Other EDs can bind to hormone receptors without activating them, thereby preventing natural hormones from binding and exerting their normal effects (Endocrine Society, n.d.).
- Alter hormone synthesis, metabolism, or transport: EDs can interfere with the production, breakdown, or transport of natural hormones, leading to abnormal hormone levels in the body (Diamanti-Kandarakis et al., 2009; NIEHS, n.d.-a).
- Change hormone receptor sensitivity: Some EDs can alter the number or sensitivity of hormone receptors on cells, changing how the body responds to its natural hormones.

Because hormones operate at very low concentrations to wield precise effects, even small disruptions caused by EDs could lead to significant health consequences, particularly during sensitive developmental periods like in utero or during puberty, but also throughout adulthood (NIEHS, n.d.-a; Gore et al., 2015).

Because these EDs are in so much of what we eat, touch, breathe, clean with, etc. the first step in protecting ourselves and our fertility is to be aware of where they are and avoid them as much as possible.

One well-known ED is Bisphenol A (BPA). BPA is used to make polycarbonate plastics (hard, clear plastics often used in food and beverage containers, though many are now "BPA-free") and epoxy resins (which line food cans to prevent corrosion and food contamination). "BPA-free" products may use other bisphenols like BPS or BPF, which are also under scrutiny for similar endocrine-disrupting properties (Rochester & Bolden, 2015; Konieczna et al., 2015). Thermal paper receipts are another common source of BPA or BPS. Aim to refuse receipts if you don't need them or choose an electronic receipt option so that you limit your exposure to BPA in thermal paper.

BPA is a well-known xenoestrogen, meaning it mimics estrogen (Konieczna et al., 2015; Pivonello et al., 2020). Exposure has been linked to various reproductive issues in women, including alterations in ovarian function, effects on egg quality, and potential impacts on hormone levels such as estradiol, follicle-stimulating hormone (FSH), and luteinizing hormone (LH) (Ehrlich et al., 2014; Pivonello et al., 2020). Some studies suggest associations between BPA exposure and conditions like Polycystic Ovary Syndrome (PCOS), endometriosis, and menstrual irregularities, though more research is needed to fully establish causality in humans (Kandaraki et al., 2011; Pivonello et al., 2020).

Another type of ED are phthalates - a group of chemicals used to make plastics more flexible and durable (often found in vinyl products like shower curtains, flooring, and some food packaging) and as solvents or stabilizers in personal care products like fragrances, lotions, cosmetics (nail polish, hair spray), and some medical devices (Meeker et al., 2009; NIEHS, n.d.-b).

Phthalates affect hormones by acting as anti-androgens (blocking testosterone effects) and may also affect estrogen and thyroid hormones (Meeker et al., 2009; Hauser & Calafat, 2005). Exposure has been seen to alter reproductive hormone levels - FSH, LH, and estradiol (Nobles et al., 2024). Some studies have linked higher phthalate exposure to menstrual cycle irregularities, longer cycles, anovulation, and reduced fecundability (the probability of conceiving within a menstrual cycle). (Hatch et al., 2008; Nobles et al., 2024; Johns et al., 2016).

Next, you've probably started to hear or read about the harm from Parabens. Some examples are methylparaben, propylparaben, butylparaben. Parabens are widely used as preservatives in cosmetics (makeup, moisturizers, shaving products), personal care products (shampoos, conditioners), pharmaceuticals, and some foods to prevent bacterial and fungal growth (Engeli et al., 2017; Endocrine Society, n.d.). A lot of products are now being made and promoted as "Paraben-free" which is a positive step in the right direction for promoting fertility health in the world's women.

Parabens can exhibit weak estrogenic activity, mimicking estrogen in the body (Golden et al., 2005; Routledge et al., 1998). Some research has suggested associations between paraben exposure and altered menstrual cycle length, changes in reproductive hormone levels, and potentially diminished ovarian reserve (Smith et al., 2013; Nishihama et al., 2016). However, the evidence in humans is still developing, and the estrogenic activity of parabens is generally considered much weaker than that of natural estrogen (Golden et al., 2005).

Next are pesticides. Some examples are organochlorines, organophosphates, and pyrethroids. They're used extensively in agriculture to protect crops from insects. Their residue can be found on conventionally grown fruits and vegetables, in contaminated water, and in some household pest control products (Mnif et al., 2011; Beyond Pesticides, 2025a). Many pesticides are known to be EDs and their use is slowly being restricted in many countries. To protect myself and my children from pesticides, I wash all our fruits and vegetables before eating and refrain from using pesticides and insecticides on my property.

There is also a group of EDs found in many household items called Per- and Polyfluoroalkyl Substances (PFAS). PFAS are a large group of man-made chemicals used to make products resistant to water, stains, and grease. They are found in non-stick cookware (though PFOA, a specific PFAS, has been largely phased out by major manufacturers), food packaging (e.g., some microwave popcorn bags, fast food wrappers), stain-resistant carpets and upholstery, waterproof apparel, some cosmetics, and firefighting foam (Environmental Working Group [EWG], 2024; NIEHS, n.d.-c). They linger in the environment and in the human body and are unable to be broken down. PFAS exposure has been associated with various adverse health outcomes, including effects on the endocrine system. Studies have linked PFAS exposure to altered menstrual cycle regularity, earlier age at menopause, and potential impacts on thyroid hormone levels and ovarian function (Bach et al., 2021; Nnabuchi & Duru, 2024). Some research also suggests links to reduced fertility and increased time to pregnancy (EWG, 2024).

Heavy Metals e.g., Lead, Mercury, Cadmium, Arsenic, are the next ED I'll touch on. We're seeing detoxes for heavy metals all over social media these days. Since I am not a medical professional, I can't advise on the efficacy of these different detoxes, but I urge you to understand where this heavy metal exposure is coming from so that you can avoid it entirely. Exposure can occur through contaminated water (e.g., old lead pipes), certain foods (e.g., mercury in some large predatory fish, arsenic in rice), industrial emissions, some paints (older homes with lead paint), and some consumer products or traditional remedies (Iavicoli et al., 2009; Centers for Disease Control and Prevention [CDC], n.d.).
Heavy metals can act as EDs by interfering with hormone synthesis, binding to hormone receptors, and causing oxidative stress, which can damage reproductive cells (Lavicoli et al., 2009; Pizzorno, 2023). Lead exposure has been linked to menstrual irregularities, reduced fertility, and adverse pregnancy outcomes. Cadmium can mimic estrogen and disrupt ovarian function. Mercury can also affect reproductive hormone levels (Pizzorno, 2023; Vahter, 2009).

The last EDs I want to cover here are retinoids. Most of the anti-wrinkle miracle creams that we see as women, everywhere we turn are made with retinoids. They do work well to reduce stubborn wrinkles. Retinoids are a class of compounds derived from Vitamin A. They are found in some skincare products (e.g., retinol, retinyl palmitate, tretinoin, isotretinoin) used for anti-aging and acne treatment. Dietary Vitamin A is essential for our bodies, but very high supplemental doses or certain prescription retinoids end up giving us excess. While dietary Vitamin A is crucial for reproduction, high systemic exposure to certain synthetic retinoids (especially oral prescription forms like isotretinoin, formerly Accutane) is known to be highly teratogenic (causing severe birth defects) and can also impact the endocrine system (Mount Sinai, n.d.). The primary concern with topical retinoids used in cosmetics is typically lower due to limited systemic absorption, but the potential for endocrine effects, especially with widespread or high-concentration use, is an area of ongoing research. High systemic levels of Vitamin A can disrupt hormonal balance. Always follow product usage guidelines and consult a healthcare provider if you have concerns, especially if trying to conceive or currently pregnant.

EDs can cause an interference with the hypothalamic-pituitary-ovarian (HPO) axis, the central control system for your menstrual cycle (Diamanti-Kandarakis et al., 2009; Gore et al., 2015). Disruptions can lead to:

- Irregular Menstrual Cycles: EDs can alter the length of the menstrual cycle, making periods unpredictable. This can be due to interference with the hormones that control follicular development, ovulation, or the luteal phase (Hatch et al., 2008; Louis et al., 2015).
- Anovulation or Oligoovulation: By mimicking or blocking hormones like estrogen, progesterone, FSH, or LH, EDs can prevent or reduce the frequency of ovulation (Kandaraki et al., 2011; Pivonello et al., 2020). This is a common cause of infertility.
- Altered Hormone Levels: Exposure to EDs can lead to imbalances in key reproductive hormones, which can manifest in various ways, including changes in menstrual flow, premenstrual symptoms, and difficulty conceiving (Nobles et al., 2024; Meeker et al., 2009).

- Impact on Egg Quality and Ovarian Reserve: Some EDs may be directly toxic to ovarian follicles or oocytes (eggs), potentially reducing egg quality or accelerating the depletion of ovarian reserve (the number of remaining eggs) (Pivonello et al., 2020; Smith et al., 2013).
- Conditions like PCOS or Endometriosis: While the causes of these conditions are multifactorial, ED exposure is being investigated as a potential contributing environmental factor due to their ability to disrupt hormonal pathways implicated in these disorders (Kandaraki et al., 2011; Louis et al., 2015).

I have a personal story of a hormone imbalance that happened to me while using Tretinoin topical cream to reduce my forehead wrinkle for a mere 30 days. The cream was doing wonders for my skin! I followed the directions and didn't experience any side effects of burning skin or purging acne breakouts. My skin was becoming softer and more supple, while the wrinkle was rising and becoming less deep set in the skin. I was very satisfied with what I saw in the mirror!

However, because I tracked my fertile signs using *TCS* method, I was able to determine that my body was gearing up to ovulate, but it was never able to complete the process. I observed my cervix beginning to open on Day 10, along with slippery egg-white mucus for the next 6 days. The mucus remained fertile, and the cervix opened slightly, but it never opened to its full circumference for ovulation.

On approximately Day 17, my body seemingly gave up trying to ovulate and the cervix closed and mucus dried. I went on to use my Mira[1] hormone monitor and never noted a progesterone rise for the remainder of that cycle. Because the progesterone didn't

---

[1] Mira Hormone Monitor: While not required for TCS method, I do use this on occasion and it's extremely informative in tracking your hormones (Progesterone, Estrogen, and Luteinizing Hormone) throughout your cycle to determine whether the reproductive system is working properly. It provides quantitative data you can bring to a medical professional if your numbers demonstrate a hormonal imbalance. https://www.miracare.com/

rise, I can confirm that I did not ovulate. This has never happened in my cycles prior to using this retinoid topical cream. Nothing else changed in my diet, exercise, or stress level. I have mentioned previously that I am not a doctor. However, this situation concerned me. My research concluded that topical retinoid creams can cause hormone disruption like what I was experiencing. Some bodies are more sensitive to these chemicals than other bodies and mine was affected by the chemical. Although I wasn't necessarily trying to conceive, I also didn't want to risk causing damage to my ovaries and not be able to conceive later if I wanted to. Disappointed with the side effects, I reluctantly stopped using Tretinoin after 30 days. My period came 4 days late that month, when I am usually extremely regular at 28 days. I was able to confirm ovulation the next month and every month going forward since discontinuing Tretinoin topical cream. While I can't say without a doubt that Tretinoin prevented me from ovulating, I can infer that it interfered with my hormones and led to an imbalance.

While it's nearly impossible to avoid all EDs, awareness and conscious choices can help minimize your exposure:

- Read Labels: Look for products labeled "BPA-free," "phthalate-free," and "paraben-free." Be aware that "BPA-free" may mean other bisphenols are used.
- Choose Glass or Stainless Steel: Opt for glass or stainless-steel containers for food storage and water bottles instead of plastic. Avoid microwaving food in plastic containers.
- Filter Your Water: Use a quality water filter certified to remove common contaminants, which may include some EDs.
- Eat Fresh, Whole Foods: Reduce reliance on processed and canned foods. Wash fruits and vegetables thoroughly to remove pesticide residues. Consider organic options when possible.

- Select Safer Personal Care Products and Cosmetics: Look for products with simpler ingredient lists and fewer synthetic chemicals. Resources like the Environmental Working Group's (EWG) Skin Deep® database can help you assess product safety. Opt for fragrance-free products or those scented with essential oils, as "fragrance" can be a proprietary blend hiding phthalates. You can download the EWG app on your phone for quick, convenient confirmation of what's safe and what's not.
- Use Natural Cleaning Products: Choose plant-based detergents and cleaning supplies or make your own using simple ingredients like vinegar and baking soda.
- Minimize Handling of Thermal Paper Receipts: Decline receipts when possible or wash your hands after handling them.
- Improve Indoor Air Quality: Dust and vacuum regularly (using a HEPA filter vacuum if possible), as some EDs can accumulate in household dust. Ventilate your home well.

Trying to immediately rid your life of all endocrine-disrupting chemicals feels hopeless and overwhelming, but knowledge empowers you to make more informed choices for your reproductive health. Make small changes over time so that the changes are manageable for you. While the science is continually evolving, there is growing evidence that exposure to certain EDs found in everyday products can interfere with the delicate hormonal balance necessary for a regular menstrual cycle and optimal fertility signs. We need our fertile signs to be accurate so that we can trust them to correctly track our cycles.

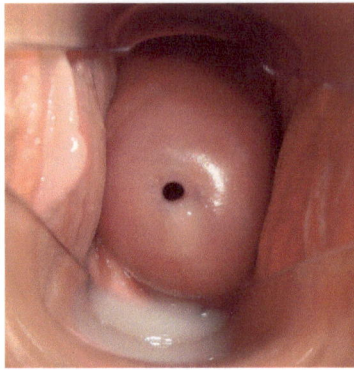

Let's Find Your Cervix!

What Supplies Are Needed:

- Your mind (for observation and learning)

- Your fingers (clean!)

- Fertility journal (or just a pen and paper/app)

- LH strips (optional but recommended for pinpointing ovulation timing)

- Progesterone test strips, Proov for example (optional, for confirming ovulation)

You will begin tracking on Day 1. Day 1 is the first day that your menstrual blood is truly flowing (not just spotting). Make note in your journal of how many days you bleed (i.e., require a pad or tampon).

How to Locate and Check Your Cervix:

1. **Wash and dry your hands thoroughly.** Ensure fingernails are short and smooth.

2. **Find a comfortable position.** Standing with one foot raised on a stool or toilet edge, or squatting, often works well. Some prefer checking in the shower. Consistency in position is key for comparable observations day-to-day.

3. **Gently insert the middle or index finger** of your dominant hand into your vagina. Aim slightly upwards and towards your back.

4. **Continue inserting until your finger meets a firmer, somewhat rounded structure** – like hitting a soft wall or the tip of a nose. This is your cervix!

5. **Gently feel the surface.** Note its texture (firm like the tip of your nose, or soft like your lips) and its position (how far did you have to reach? Low, medium, or high?).

6. **Locate the opening (os).** Feel for a small dimple, slit, or hole in the center. Note whether it feels closed (like a dimple), slightly open (like a slit), or more open (can perhaps fit the tip of your finger slightly inside). The shape and size of the os can vary between women, especially those who have given birth vaginally, will have a wider, almost always slightly open os due to it being widened for childbirth.

7. **Withdraw your finger and observe any cervical mucus.** Note its color (clear, white, yellowish), consistency (dry, sticky, creamy, watery, stretchy like egg white), and amount.

8. **Record your findings** in your journal/app: Cycle Day, Cervix Position (Low/Medium/High), Cervix Texture (Firm/Soft), Cervix Opening (Closed/Slightly Open/Open), Mucus characteristics.

9. **Check consistently,** ideally once a day, around the same time. Avoid checking immediately after intercourse, as semen can obscure mucus observations.

If you have trouble finding your cervix initially, don't get discouraged! Try again the next day or in a different position. It takes practice.

Making Sense of Your Cervix & Mucus:

FERTILE DAYS: Fertile days encompass the time leading up to and including ovulation. This is when conception is possible. Sperm can survive in fertile cervical mucus for up to 5 days (Cleveland Clinic, n.d.-b; Taunton et al., 2014), while the egg is viable for about 12-24 hours after ovulation (Cleveland Clinic, n.d.-b). Therefore, the "fertile window" typically starts several days *before* ovulation occurs.

Signs indicating increasing fertility and approaching ovulation include:

- Cervix becoming higher, softer, and more open (myFertileDays, n.d.; Reed & Carr, 2024).

- Cervical mucus becoming more abundant, clearer, wetter, and stretchier (like raw egg white) (Leão & Esteves, 2024; myFertileDays, n.d.; Taunton et al., 2014).

To pinpoint ovulation more precisely, you can use LH strips in addition to cervical observations. Begin using LH strips daily starting a few days after your period ends (or based on your typical cycle length). Follow the package instructions. A positive LH test indicates the LH surge is occurring, and ovulation is likely to happen within the next 24-36 hours (Reed & Carr, 2024).

You should find that around the time of a positive LH test, your cervix feels high, soft, and maximally open, accompanied by abundant, slippery, egg-white mucus. This peak fertility state typically lasts around the day of ovulation.

About 24-48 hours after ovulation (post-LH surge), you should notice the cervix beginning to lower, firm up, and close, and mucus becoming less abundant, thicker, and stickier (myFertileDays, n.d.; Reed & Carr, 2024). Observing this distinct shift helps confirm the fertile window is closing.

Checking morning and evening during this transition time can help you clearly identify the change.

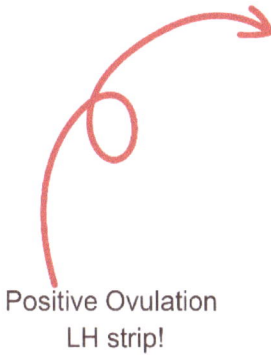

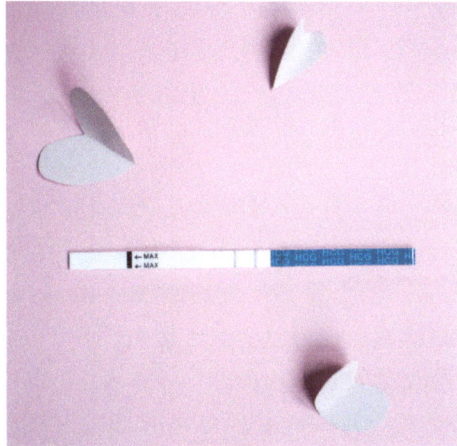

Positive Ovulation LH strip!

IMPORTANT: If you experience extended periods of fertile-quality mucus and an open/soft/high cervix *without* a subsequent shift to infertile signs (closed/firm/low cervix, dry/sticky mucus), ovulation may be delayed. Continue to consider yourself fertile as long as fertile signs persist, regardless of passing the calculated "Day 14". Stress, illness, travel, or other factors can delay ovulation (Cleveland Clinic, n.d.-b; Medical News Today, 2024).

Here's my real-life example: During a trip to San Diego for a conference, despite expecting ovulation on the day I left based on my fertile mucus and opening cervix, my cervix remained high, soft, half-way open, and wet throughout the 3-day trip. The shift to fully open and then infertile signs only occurred after I returned home, indicating delayed ovulation likely due to travel stress. Relying on my current cervical signs, not just predictions, was crucial.

To *confirm* ovulation occurred, you can use progesterone test strips (like Proov) starting about 5-7 days after your suspected ovulation day (or follow package instructions). These detect the rise in progesterone metabolite (PdG) that occurs *after* ovulation

(Mayo Clinic, 2023; StatPearls, n.d.-a). A positive result confirms ovulation likely occurred. If you consistently see fertile signs (mucus, open cervix) but do not get a positive progesterone test result month after month, you might be experiencing anovulatory cycles (cycles without ovulation) and should consult a healthcare provider, bringing your tracking data.

INFERTILE DAYS: Infertile days occur *after* ovulation is confirmed by the shift back to infertile signs (low, firm, closed cervix and dry or sticky/creamy mucus) and potentially a positive progesterone test. This post-ovulatory infertile phase (luteal phase) typically lasts 10-16 days until your next period begins. During this confirmed infertile phase, pregnancy is highly unlikely. Sometimes this is referred to as "Phase 3."

IMPORTANT NOTE ON PRE-OVULATORY PHASE: The days immediately following menstruation *before* fertile signs appear are questionable days. You may not have begun experiencing signs of fertility; however, sperm *can* survive in the Fallopian tubes for several days (Cleveland Clinic, n.d.-b; Taunton et al., 2014). If you have intercourse during these early "dry days" and then ovulate earlier than expected, conception *is* possible. Therefore, if strictly avoiding pregnancy, these early cycle days before the clear shift *to* fertile signs may not be reliably "safe" without using a barrier method or abstaining. The safest infertile time for avoiding pregnancy is the confirmed post-ovulatory phase.

Practice Makes Perfect: Observe and chart your cervical signs and mucus daily for approximately 3 months to become familiar with *your* unique pattern: when you typically ovulate, how long your cycles are, and what your specific fertile vs. non-fertile signs feel and look like.

QUICK RECAP of TCS Method Data Points:

- Day Period Began (Day 1)

- Day Period Ended

- Daily Cervix Check:

    - Position (High/Medium/Low)

    - Texture (Soft/Firm)

    - Opening (Open/Slightly Open/Closed)

- Daily Mucus Check:

    - Consistency (Dry/Sticky/Creamy/Watery/Egg white)

    - Sensation (Dry/Damp/Wet/Slippery)

    - Color (Clear/Cloudy/White/Yellowish)

- LH Test Result (Optional: Positive/Negative)

- Progesterone Test Result (Optional: Positive/Negative)

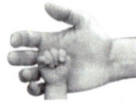

TO ACHIEVE PREGNANCY: Plan intercourse during your fertile window. Start having intercourse every 1-2 days once you notice the beginning of fertile signs (mucus becoming thin/stretchy, cervix starting to soften/rise/open). Continue through the day of peak signs (most fertile mucus, highest/softest/most open cervix) and potentially the day after. Using LH strips can help time intercourse closer to ovulation.

OPEN CERVIX + FERTILE MUCUS = PRIME TIME TO TTC

Remember, your fertile window timing may vary month to month, so rely on your *current* signs.

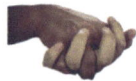

TO PREVENT PREGNANCY: Avoid unprotected intercourse during your entire fertile window. The fertile window begins with the *first* sign of fertile mucus or cervical changes indicating approaching ovulation. It ends *only after* ovulation has been confirmed by a clear and sustained shift back to infertile signs (low/firm/closed cervix AND dry/sticky mucus) for at least 3 consecutive days. To be extra conservative, wait until the evening of the 3rd day *after* the peak fertile signs (or the 4th day of the temperature rise if using BBT) before considering yourself in the infertile phase. Using progesterone strips to confirm ovulation adds another layer of certainty. The confirmed post-ovulatory phase, is the safest time for unprotected intercourse if avoiding pregnancy. Do *not* rely on early cycle "dry days" as completely safe. Abstinence or using barrier methods during the entire potentially fertile period is necessary for high effectiveness in preventing pregnancy.

CLOSED CERVIX + NO MUCUS + OVULATION CONFIRMED = PRIME TIME TO TTA

Integrating *The Cervical Solution* into Your Life

If you are not currently using hormonal birth control, you can begin tracking your signs immediately. Start by noting the day of your cycle and recording your daily cervical and mucus observations.

If you are transitioning off hormonal birth control, be aware that it can take time for your true cycle and fertility signs to regulate and become reliable. This period varies significantly depending on the method used and the individual. For pills, patches, rings, IUDs, and implants, fertility often returns within 1-3 months, though it can take longer for cycles to fully normalize (Girum & Wasie, 2018; Verywell Health, 2025; Yland et al., 2020). For injectable contraceptives (like Depo-Provera), the return to ovulation and fertility can be significantly delayed, sometimes taking 6-12 months or even longer (Girum & Wasie, 2018; Verywell Health, 2025). During this transition phase, your observed signs may be inconsistent or misleading. It's advisable to use a reliable barrier method or abstain if avoiding pregnancy, until you observe several consistent, predictable cycles that align with the patterns described in this book. Consulting a healthcare provider knowledgeable about FAMs during this transition can also be helpful.

A key part of successfully using *TCS* (or any FAM) is ensuring your partner is informed and supportive, if you're in a relationship. Discuss your goals (achieving or avoiding pregnancy) and how you will use your observations to guide decisions about intimacy. Open communication, mutual respect, and understanding are essential, especially during the learning phase or transition periods. It might take time for both of you to adjust, but the benefits of understanding and working with your natural cycle can strengthen your connection and empower you both.

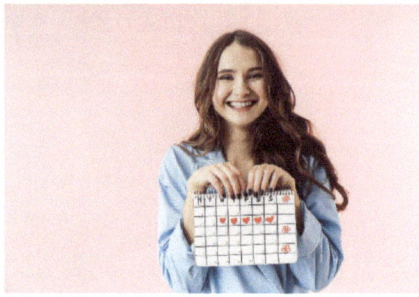

Embracing Your Unique Fertility Story

Choosing to understand your reproductive system through fertility awareness is not to be taken lightly. It can feel daunting, confusing, or frustrating at times, especially initially. I understand; I've been there! Know that you are NOT alone. Many women are on similar journeys. Support each other! Your body is not weird or broken. Be patient with yourself. You CAN do this!

It requires dedication, especially at first, to perform daily checks, record findings, and analyze patterns over several cycles. But once you become attuned to your body's rhythms – how your cervix moves, how your mucus changes – you will gain a clear understanding of your personal fertile and non-fertile times. This learning process might take months, or perhaps longer, up to a year for some, especially if cycles are irregular or transitioning. This investment of time is actually small compared to the lifelong knowledge, confidence, and empowerment you will gain.

The fertility you possess is a significant part of being female. With the knowledge gained from observing your body, using your cervix and its mucus as guides, you can make informed decisions aligned with your reproductive goals. This understanding can foster strength and respect for your body and its capabilities. Consider passing this vital information on to future generations, empowering both women and men to make informed choices about reproductive health, moving beyond solely relying on artificial and often harmful birth control methods.

If I can be of any assistance, please don't hesitate to reach me on my website **www.thepursuitoffertility.com** or via email at thepursuitoffertility@gmail.com. I founded The Pursuit of Fertility to provide both fertility awareness coaching and perinatal grief support to women. I can help you once, twice, or as many times as you need it, to get you confident in using your own body to achieve or prevent pregnancy. I offer pay-what-you-can services because I wholeheartedly believe in helping others in need and spreading body literacy education. I wish you all the best on your natural fertility journey using *The Cervical Solution*!

References

American College of Obstetricians and Gynecologists (ACOG). (2021). *Alcohol and women*. https://www.acog.org/womens-health/faqs/alcohol-and-women

Bach, C. C., Bodin, J., Bølling, A. K., Eljarrat, E., Fingerhut, A., Gyllenhammar, I., ... & Vinnars, B. (2021). *Perfluoroalkyl substances (PFAS) in the Nordic countries: Occurrence, fate, and MATE-effects*. Nordic Council of Ministers. https://pub.norden.org/temanord2021-507/

Better Health Channel. (2020). *Weight, fertility and pregnancy health*. https://www.betterhealth.vic.gov.au/health/conditionsandtreatments/weight-fertility-and-pregnancy-health

Beyond Pesticides. (2025, April 8). Literature review of over 200 studies highlights pesticide threats to women's reproductive health. *Beyond Pesticides Daily News Blog*. https://beyondpesticides.org/dailynewsblog/2025/04/literature-review-of-over-200-studies-highlights-pesticide-threats-to-womens-reproductive-health/

Boston University. (2020, November 16). When does fertility return after stopping contraceptive use? *SPH News*. https://www.bu.edu/sph/news/articles/2020/when-does-fertility-return-after-stopping-contraceptive-use/

Bretveld, R. W., Thomas, C. M. G., Scheepers, P. T. J., Zielhuis, G. A., & Roeleveld, N. (2006). Pesticide exposure: The hormonal function of the female reproductive system disrupted? *Reproductive Biology and Endocrinology*, *4*, 30. https://doi.org/10.1186/1477-7827-4-30

Centers for Disease Control and Prevention (CDC). (n.d.). *About lead and other heavy metals and reproductive health*. National Institute for Occupational Safety and Health. Retrieved May 15, 2025, from https://www.cdc.gov/niosh/reproductive-health/prevention/lead-metals.html

Cleveland Clinic. (n.d.-a). *Basal body temperature: Family planning method*. Retrieved May 4, 2025, from https://my.clevelandclinic.org/health/articles/21065-basal-body-temperature

Cleveland Clinic. (n.d.-b). *Cervical mucus: Chart, stages, tracking & fertility*. Retrieved May 15, 2025, from https://my.clevelandclinic.org/health/body/21957-cervical-mucus

Cleveland Clinic. (n.d.-c). *Rhythm method: Birth control, calendar & effectiveness*. Retrieved May 4, 2025, from https://my.clevelandclinic.org/health/articles/17900-rhythm-method

Cleveland Clinic. (2022, June 15). *Cervix: Anatomy, function, changes & conditions*. https://my.clevelandclinic.org/health/body/23279-cervix

Diamanti-Kandarakis, E., Bourguignon, J. P., Giudice, L. C., Hauser, R., Prins, G. S., Soto, A. M., ... & Gore, A. C. (2009). Endocrine-disrupting chemicals: An Endocrine Society scientific statement. *Endocrine Reviews, 30*(4), 293–342. https://doi.org/10.1210/er.2009-0002

Ehrlich, S., Williams, P. L., Missmer, S. A., Flaws, J. A., Ye, X., Calafat, A. M., ... & Hauser, R. (2014). Urinary bisphenol A concentrations and association with ovarian reserve among women from a fertility clinic. *Human Reproduction, 29*(2), 359–366. https://doi.org/10.1093/humrep/det429

Endocrine Society. (n.d.). *Endocrine-disrupting chemicals (EDCs)*. Retrieved May 15, 2025, from https://www.endocrine.org/patient-engagement/endocrine-library/edcs

Engeli, R. T., Rohrer, S. R., Vuorinen, A., Herdlinger, S., Kaserer, T., Leugger, S. T., ... & Odermatt, A. (2017). Interference of paraben compounds with estrogen metabolism by inhibition of 17β-hydroxysteroid dehydrogenases. *International Journal of Molecular Sciences*, *18*(9), 2007. https://doi.org/10.3390/ijms18092007

Environmental Working Group (EWG). (2024, March). *PFAS and developmental and reproductive toxicity: An EWG fact sheet*. https://www.ewg.org/news-insights/news/2024/03/pfas-and-developmental-and-reproductive-toxicity-ewg-fact-sheet

Fisher, S. (2020, January 24). *Natural Family Planning can be hard (and expensive) to use. Can new tech help?* America Magazine. https://www.americamagazine.org/faith/2020/01/24/natural-family-planning-can-be-hard-and-expensive-use-can-new-tech-help

Gaskins, A. J., & Chavarro, J. E. (2018). Diet and fertility: A review. *American Journal of Obstetrics and Gynecology*, *218*(4), 379–389. https://doi.org/10.1016/j.ajog.2017.08.010

Genesis OBGYN. (n.d.). *Dear Doctor: Should I get fit to prepare for pregnancy?* Retrieved May 15, 2025, from https://genesisobgyn.net/getting-fit-how-to-prepare-for-pregnancy/

Girum, T., & Wasie, A. (2018). Return of fertility after discontinuation of contraception: a systematic review and meta-analysis. *Contraception and Reproductive Medicine*, *3*, 9. https://contraceptionmedicine.biomedcentral.com/articles/10.1186/s40834-018-0064-y

Golden, R., Gandy, J., & Vollmer, G. (2005). A review of the endocrine activity of parabens and implications for potential risks to human health. *Critical Reviews in Toxicology*, *35*(5), 435–458. https://doi.org/10.1080/10408440490920104

Gore, A. C., Chappell, V. A., Fenton, S. E., Flaws, J. A., Nadal, A., Prins, G. S., ... & Zoeller, R. T. (2015). EDC-2: The Endocrine Society's second scientific statement on endocrine-disrupting chemicals. *Endocrine Reviews*, *36*(6), E1–E150. https://doi.org/10.1210/er.2015-1010

Hatch, E. E., Nelson, J. W., Qureshi, M. M., Weinberg, J., Moore, L. L., Singer, M., & Shalat, S. L. (2008). Association of urinary phthalate metabolite concentrations with body mass index and waist circumference: A cross-sectional study of NHANES data, 1999-2002. *Environmental Health*, *7*, 27. https://doi.org/10.1186/1476-069X-7-27

Hauser, R., & Calafat, A. M. (2005). Phthalates and human health. *Occupational and Environmental Medicine*, *62*(11), 806–818. https://doi.org/10.1136/oem.2004.017590

Iavicoli, I., Fontana, L., & Bergamaschi, A. (2009). The effects of metals as endocrine disruptors. *Journal of Toxicology and Environmental Health, Part B*, *12*(3), 206–223. https://doi.org/10.1080/10937400902902067

Johns, L. E., Cooper, G. S., Galizia, A., & Meeker, J. D. (2016). Exposure to phthalates and feminine reproductive health. *Current Epidemiology Reports*, *3*(2), 135–147. https://doi.org/10.1007/s40471-016-0072-y

Jurewicz, J., Radwan, M., Wielgomas, B., Kałużny, P., Klimowska, A., Radwan, P., ... & Hanke, W. (2017). Environmental exposure to triclosan and female fertility. *International Journal of Environmental Research and Public Health*, *14*(10), 1146. https://doi.org/10.3390/ijerph14101146

Kandaraki, E., Chatzigeorgiou, A., Livadas, S., Palioura, E., Economou, F., Koutsilieris, M., ... & Diamanti-Kandarakis, E. (2011). Endocrine disruptors and Polycystic Ovary Syndrome (PCOS): A plethora of potential molecular mechanisms. *Therapeutic Advances in Endocrinology and Metabolism*, *2*(6), 249–274. https://doi.org/10.1177/2042018811430219

Kesmodel, U., Olsen, J., & Schønheyder, H. C. (2002). Does moderate alcohol consumption affect fertility? Follow up study among couples planning first pregnancy. *BMJ*, *325*(7371), 1049. https://doi.org/10.1136/bmj.325.7371.1049

Konieczna, A., Rutkowska, A., & Rachoń, D. (2015). Health risk of exposure to Bisphenol A (BPA). *Roczniki Państwowego Zakładu Higieny*, *66*(1), 5–11.

Lancaster General Health. (2022, October). *Fertility and your weight: How they're connected*. https://www.lancastergeneralhealth.org/health-hub-home/2022/october/fertility-and-your-weight-how-theyre-connected

Leão, R. B. F., & Esteves, S. C. (2015). Insights into the role of cervical mucus and vaginal pH in unexplained infertility. *MedicalExpress (São Paulo, online)*, *11*, e20240101. https://www.scielo.br/j/medical/a/qjRg5mV765Dvs5tYjCtBwyC/

Louis, G. M. B., Peterson, C. M., Chen, Z., Croughan, M., Sundaram, R., Stanford, J., ... & Buck Louis, G. M. (2015). Environmental PCB exposure and risk of endometriosis. *Human Reproduction*, *30*(1), 199–207. https://doi.org/10.1093/humrep/deu289

Maher, R. A., Wadden, K., Fuller, D., Basset, F., & Murphy, H. (2023). The current landscape of exercise and female fertility research: a narrative review in exercise prescription. *Reproduction*, *165*(5), R69–R82. https://doi.org/10.1530/REP-22-0317

Mayo Clinic. (2023, February 10). *Basal body temperature for natural family planning*. https://www.mayoclinic.org/tests-procedures/basal-body-temperature/about/pac-20393026

Medical News Today. (2024, March 7). *Fertility awareness method: Effectiveness for birth control.* https://www.medicalnewstoday.com/articles/how-effective-is-fertility-awareness

Meeker, J. D., Sathyanarayana, S., & Swan, S. H. (2009). Phthalates and other additives in plastics: Human exposure and associated health outcomes. *Philosophical Transactions of the Royal Society B: Biological Sciences*, *364*(1526), 2097–2113. https://doi.org/10.1098/rstb.2008.0268

Mnif, W., Hassine, A. I. H., Bouaziz, A., Bartegi, A., Thomas, O., & Roig, B. (2011). Effect of endocrine disruptor pesticides: A review. *International Journal of Environmental Research and Public Health*, *8*(6), 2265–2303. https://doi.org/10.3390/ijerph8062265

Mount Sinai. (n.d.). *Vitamin A (Retinol)*. Health Library. Retrieved May 15, 2025, from https://www.mountsinai.org/health-library/supplement/vitamin-a-retinol

myFertileDays. (n.d.). *The phases of the menstrual cycle and associated physiological changes*. Retrieved May 4, 2025, from http://www.myfertiledays.com/en/content/phases-menstrual-cycle-and-associated-physiological-changes

National Health Service. (2024, March 11). *Natural family planning*. https://www.nhs.uk/contraception/methods-of-contraception/natural-family-planning/

National Institute of Environmental Health Sciences (NIEHS). (n.d.-a). *Endocrine disruptors*. Retrieved May 15, 2025, from https://www.niehs.nih.gov/health/topics/agents/endocrine/index.cfm

National Institute of Environmental Health Sciences (NIEHS). (n.d.-b). *Perfluoroalkyl and Polyfluoroalkyl Substances (PFAS)*. Retrieved May 15, 2025, from https://www.niehs.nih.gov/health/topics/agents/pfas/index.cfm

National Institute of Environmental Health Sciences (NIEHS). (n.d.-c). *Phthalates*. Retrieved May 15, 2025, from https://www.niehs.nih.gov/health/topics/agents/phthalates/index.cfm

Nishihama, Y., Yoshinaga, J., Iida, A., Konishi, S., Imai, H., Yoneyama, M., ... & Saito, S. (2016). Association between paraben exposure and menstrual cycle in female university students in Japan. *Reproductive Toxicology, 63*, 107–113. https://doi.org/10.1016/j.reprotox.2016.05.011

Nnabuchi, M., & Duru, C. (2024). PFAS toxicity and female reproductive health: A review of the evidence and current state of knowledge. *Substantia, 10*(1), 109-121. https://doi.org/10.36253/Substantia-2842

Nobles, C. J., Mendola, P., Kim, K., Männistö, T., Sundaram, R., Thoma, M. E., ... & Schisterman, E. F. (2024). Preconception phthalate exposure and women's reproductive health: Pregnancy, pregnancy loss, and underlying mechanisms. *Environmental Health Perspectives, 132*(1), 017001. https://doi.org/10.1289/EHP12287

Ovum Fertility. (n.d.). *How sedentary lifestyle affects fertility*. Retrieved May 15, 2025, from https://ovumfertility.in/effects-of-sedentary-lifestyle-on-fertility/

Panth, N., Gavarkovs, A., Tamez, M., & Mattei, J. (2018). The influence of diet on fertility and the implications for public health nutrition in the United States. *Frontiers in Public Health, 6*, 211. https://doi.org/10.3389/fpubh.2018.00211

Pivonello, C., Muscogiuri, G., Nardone, A., Garifalos, F., Calogero, A. E., Graziadio, C., ... & Colao, A. (2020). Bisphenol A: An emerging threat to female fertility. *Reproductive Biology and Endocrinology*, *18*, 22. https://doi.org/10.1186/s12958-020-00579-w

Pizzorno, J. (2023). Canaries in the coal mine: The impact of common environmental toxins on human reproduction. *Integrative Medicine (Encinitas, Calif.)*, *22*(1), 12–21.

Reed, B. G., & Carr, B. R. (2024). Physiology, menstrual cycle. In *StatPearls*. StatPearls Publishing. https://www.ncbi.nlm.nih.gov/books/NBK500020/

Reproductive Science Center. (n.d.). *How to build a fertility enhancing diet*. Retrieved May 15, 2025, from https://rscbayarea.com/article/build-fertility-enhancing-diet/

Reproductive Science Center of New Jersey. (n.d.). *The link between exercise and fertility*. Retrieved May 15, 2025, from https://fertilitynj.com/blog/link-between-exercise-and-fertility/

Rochester, J. R., & Bolden, A. L. (2015). Bisphenol S and F: A systematic review and comparison of the hormonal activity of bisphenol A substitutes. *Environmental Health Perspectives*, *123*(7), 643–650. https://doi.org/10.1289/ehp.1408989

Routledge, E. J., Parker, J., Odum, J., Ashby, J., & Sumpter, J. P. (1998). Some alkyl hydroxy benzoate preservatives (parabens) are estrogenic. *Toxicology and Applied Pharmacology*, *153*(1), 12–19. https://doi.org/10.1006/taap.1998.8544

Singh, S., Kaur, P., & Bala, R. (2018). A study on effectiveness of lactational amenorrhea as a method of contraception. *International Journal of Reproduction, Contraception, Obstetrics and Gynecology*, *7*(9), 3596–3600. https://www.ijrcog.org/index.php/ijrcog/article/view/5512/3866

Smith, K. W., Souter, I., Dimitriadis, I., Ehrlich, S., Williams, P. L., Calafat, A. M., & Hauser, R. (2013). Urinary paraben concentrations and ovarian aging among women from a fertility center. *Environmental Health Perspectives, 121*(11-12), 1299–1305. https://doi.org/10.1289/ehp.1205350

StatPearls. (n.d.). *Physiology, ovulation and basal body temperature*. Retrieved May 4, 2025, from https://www.ncbi.nlm.nih.gov/books/NBK546686/

Stoker, T. E., Gibson, E. K., & Zorrilla, L. M. (2010). Triclosan exposure modulates estrogen-dependent responses in the female Wistar rat. *Toxicological Sciences, 117*(1), 45–53. https://doi.org/10.1093/toxsci/kfq180

Stony Brook Medicine. (n.d.). *Drink up during the summer: The importance of hydration*. Island Fertility. Retrieved May 15, 2025, from https://www.stonybrookmedicine.edu/islandfertility/news/hydration

Taunton, C., D'Costa, Z. J., Flanagan, A. M., & Fofaria, M. M. (2014). Role of the cervix in fertility: is it time for a reappraisal? *Human Reproduction, 29*(10), 2092–2098. https://pubmed.ncbi.nlm.nih.gov/25069501/

Texas Fertility Center. (n.d.). *The basics of caffeine and fertility*. Retrieved May 15, 2025, from https://txfertility.com/blog/the-basics-of-caffeine-and-fertility/

U.S. Food and Drug Administration (FDA). (2016, September 6). *FDA issues final rule on safety and effectiveness of antibacterial soaps*. [Press release]. https://www.fda.gov/news-events/press-announcements/fda-issues-final-rule-safety-and-effectiveness-antibacterial-soaps

UC Davis Health. (2023, September 13). *This postpartum contraception is more effective than condoms or birth control pills*. https://health.ucdavis.edu/news/headlines/this-postpartum-contraception-is-more-effective-than-condoms-or-birth-control-pills/2023/09

UNC School of Medicine. (n.d.). *Cervical mucus monitoring | Time to conceive*. Retrieved May 4, 2025, from https://www.med.unc.edu/timetoconceive/study-participant-resources/cervical-mucus-testing-information/

Uni ScholarWorks. (n.d.). *The effects of exercise-induced amenorrhea on the fertility of female athletes*. Retrieved May 15, 2025, from https://scholarworks.uni.edu/cgi/viewcontent.cgi?article=5320&context=grp

Vahter, M. (2009). Effects of arsenic on maternal and fetal health. *Annual Review of Nutrition*, *29*, 381–399. https://doi.org/10.1146/annurev-nutr-080508-141102

Van der Wijden, C., & Manheimer, E. (1998). Postpartum contraception: the lactational amenorrhea method. *European Journal of Contraception & Reproductive Health Care*, *3*(2), 91-102. https://pubmed.ncbi.nlm.nih.gov/9678098/

Verywell Health. (2025, February 28). *When does fertility return after stopping birth control?* https://www.verywellhealth.com/when-does-fertility-return-after-stopping-birth-control-4056322

Weatherly, L. M., & Gosse, J. A. (2017). Triclosan exposure, transformation, and human health effects. *Journal of Toxicology and Environmental Health, Part B*, *20*(8), 447–469. https://doi.org/10.1080/10937404.2017.1399306

Yland, J. J., Jukic, A. M. Z., Hatch, E. E., Rothman, K. J., Sørensen, H. T., Riis, A. H., Wesselink, A. K., Huybrechts, K. F., & Wise, L. A. (2020). Pregravid contraceptive use and fecundability: a prospective cohort study. *BMJ, 371*, m3966. https://www.bmj.com/content/371/bmj.m3966.long

Your Fertility. (2018). *Caffeine.* https://www.yourfertility.org.au/everyone/drugs-chemicals/caffeine

Zorrilla, L. M., Gibson, E. K., Jeffay, S. C., Crofton, K. M., Setzer, W. R., Cooper, R. L., & Stoker, T. E. (2009). The effects of triclosan on puberty and thyroid hormones in male Wistar rats. *Toxicological Sciences, 107*(1), 56–64. https://doi.org/10.1093/toxsci/kfn225

Index

F

G

H

I

L

M